BODY WORKS™

GUTS

The Digestive System

Gillian Houghton

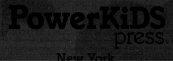

PowerKiDS press.

New York

Published in 2007 by The Rosen Publishing Group, Inc.
29 East 21st Street, New York, NY 10010

First Edition

Editors: Daryl Heller and Amelie von Zumbusch
Book Design: Greg Tucker

Photo Credits: Cover © 3D Clinic/Getty Images; p. 5 © Superstock, Inc./Superstock; p. 6 (top) © Photodisc; p. 6 (bottom) © age
fotostock/Superstock; p. 9 © USDA Center For Nutrition Policy and Promotion; p. 10 (top) © Eyewire; p. 10 (bottom) © John
Karapelou,CMI/Phototake; p. 13 (left) © Sophie Jacopin/Photo Researchers, Inc; p. 13(right) © Ricky John Molloy/Getty Images; pp. 14, 21 ©
Anatomical Travelogue/Photo Researchers, Inc; p. 17 (left) © James Cavallini/Photo Researchers, Inc; p. 17 (right) © Bo Veisland, MI&I/Photo
Researchers, Inc; p. 18 (left) © SPL/Photo Researchers, Inc; p. 18 (right) © John M. Daugherty/Photo Researchers, Inc.

Library of Congress Cataloging-in-Publication Data

Houghton, Gillian.
  Guts : the digestive system / Gillian Houghton.
      p. cm. — (Body works)
  Includes index.
  ISBN (10) 1-4042-3470-5 (13) 978-1-4042-3470-3 (lib. bdg.) — ISBN (10) 1-4042-2179-4 (13) 978-1-4042-2179-6 (pbk.)
  1. Digestive organs—Juvenile literature. 2. Digestion—Juvenile literature. I. Title. II. Series.
  QP145.H68 2007
  612.3—dc22
                                    2005032934

Manufactured in the United States of America

Contents

The Digestive System 4

Eat Your Energy! 7

What Is on Your Plate? 8

The Mouth 11

A Closer Look at the Teeth 12

Swallow! 15

The Esophagus and the Stomach 16

The Intestines 19

The Big Glands 20

Digestive Trouble 22

Glossary 23

Index 24

Web Sites 24

The Digestive System

The digestive system is made up of body parts that help turn the food you eat into the power your body needs. The digestive system is a long tunnel of **muscle**. As food passes through this tunnel, it mixes with digestive juices. Digestive juices are made up of special **proteins**, **acids**, and salts. They help digest, or break down, food. When food is digested, **nutrients** and water are taken in by the inside walls of some parts of the digestive system. The matter that cannot be taken in leaves the body as waste.

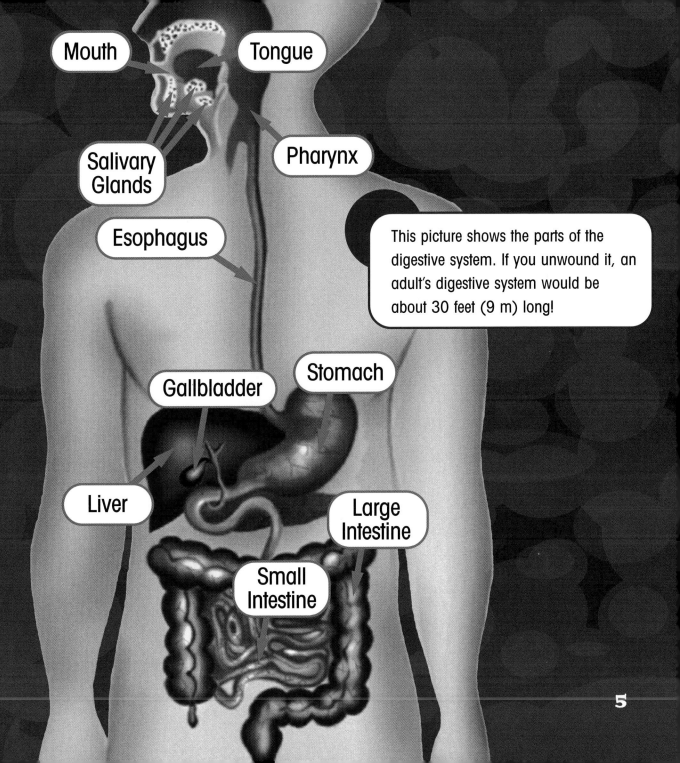

Mouth

Tongue

Salivary Glands

Pharynx

Esophagus

This picture shows the parts of the digestive system. If you unwound it, an adult's digestive system would be about 30 feet (9 m) long!

Stomach

Gallbladder

Liver

Large Intestine

Small Intestine

People get the energy their bodies need from the food that they eat. Vegetables and fruits, like tomatoes, have many of the nutrients the body needs.

Eat Your Energy!

As food is digested, energy is given off. Energy is the power to work or act. Food's energy is measured in **calories**. One small bowl of carrots has about 25 calories. A piece of bread with butter has 125 calories. Energy-rich foods are good to eat, but higher-calorie foods are not always better for you. A glass of low-fat milk has 120 calories. A can of soda has 150 calories. Milk is still healthier for you. It is made up of the stuff your body needs to play, work, and grow.

What Is on Your Plate?

Food is made up of **carbohydrates**, fats, proteins, **vitamins**, **minerals**, and water. Carbohydrates are found in bread, rice, and vegetables. During digestion carbohydrates break down into sugars. Sugars give your body energy. Fats are found in eggs and oils. They help the body stay warm and store energy. Proteins are found in meats and beans. Proteins break down into acids that keep your bones and muscles strong. The body can take in vitamins, minerals, and water just as they are. Vitamins help the body fight illness. Minerals such as calcium help build bones.

The U.S. government suggests how much people should eat based on things such as how old a person is and how much exercise that person gets. This pyramid shows how much the government thinks a ten-year-old who gets 30 to 60 minutes of exercise each day should eat in one day.

GRAINS **VEGETABLES** **FRUITS** **MILK** **MEAT & BEANS**

6 ounces
A piece of bread is about 1 ounce. Bread, rolls, rice, and pasta are all grains.

2.5 cups
Peas, carrots, and squash are some of the many choices in the vegetable group.

1.5 cups
Apples, strawberries, and grapes are all fruits. Fruit juices are also a form of fruit.

3 cups
The milk group includes not only milk, but also cheese and yogurt.

5 ounces
Chicken, fish, peanut butter, steak, and tofu are all part of the meat & beans group.

Your tongue helps you swallow. It also lets you taste your food.

Teeth

Salivary Glands

Tongue

The Mouth

The digestive system begins with the mouth. Lips help pull food into the mouth. Teeth tear food into bites. The **tongue** and **jaw** move food from side to side. The tongue is a group of muscles fixed to the bottom of the mouth. The top and bottom bones of the jaw form a base for the teeth. Teeth come together to chew the food. A **liquid** in the mouth, called saliva, wets the food. This makes the food easier to swallow. A protein in saliva begins to break down food. Saliva is made by the six main salivary **glands** around the mouth.

A Closer Look at the Teeth

A healthy mouth in an adult has 32 teeth. Every tooth is made up of a root, a neck, and a crown. The root is the part of a tooth that is tied to the jaw. A tooth's neck is hidden below the gums. The gums are the firm, red inside wall of the mouth at the base of the teeth. The crown is the part of a tooth that can be seen above the gums. A strong coating called enamel covers the crown. The soft inside of a tooth is called pulp.

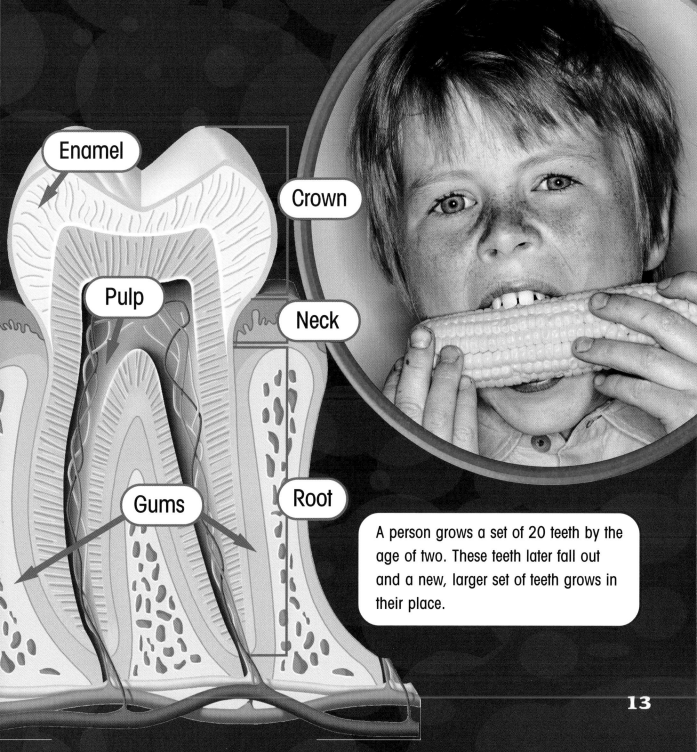

Enamel

Crown

Pulp

Neck

Gums

Root

A person grows a set of 20 teeth by the age of two. These teeth later fall out and a new, larger set of teeth grows in their place.

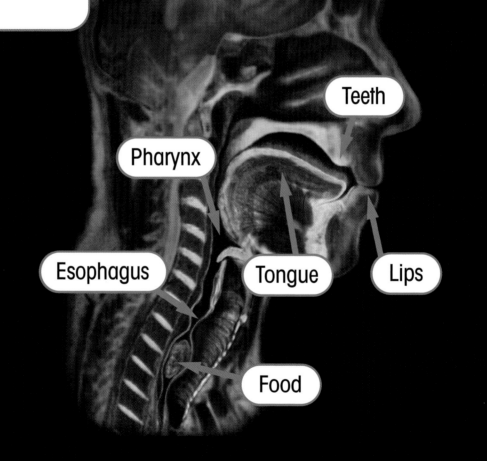

Your tongue moves food from your mouth to your pharynx. Your pharynx then pushes together to push the food toward your stomach.

Teeth

Pharynx

Esophagus

Tongue

Lips

Food

Swallow!

After a mouthful of food is chewed and coated with saliva, the tongue pushes against the top of the mouth. This moves the ball of chewed food toward the **pharynx**. The pharynx is a narrow opening at the back of the mouth. The muscles of the pharynx contract, or press together, in a wave. These contractions push the food along. A small muscle closes the tunnel that connects, or ties, the mouth and the **lungs**. Breathing stops for a short time. These movements and contractions form the action of swallowing.

The Esophagus and the Stomach

Chewed food travels through the pharynx and into the **esophagus**. The esophagus connects the pharynx and the stomach. The muscles inside the esophagus contract to push the food toward the stomach. The stomach is shaped like the letter *J*. Its inside wall is lined with millions, or thousands of thousands, of glands. These glands make **gastric juice**, which has special proteins and acids that break down and digest food. Food is stored in the stomach for about 4 hours. Then it is slowly released, or let go of, into the small intestine.

The esophagus is the
tunnel at the top of the
stomach in the
drawing above.
Inset: This picture is an
X-ray of the stomach.
An X-ray is a picture
taken with a special
tool that can see inside
the body.

The intestines lie below the stomach. The large intestine bends around the folded-up small intestine. *Inset:* The bumps on the inside of the small intestine's walls are .01 to .03 inches (.3–.8 mm) high.

The Intestines

The last steps of digestion take place in the small intestine. The small intestine is a long, narrow tunnel of muscle. It is uneven and covered with small, fingerlike bumps. These bumps are covered with even smaller bumps. The small intestine could not absorb, or take in, as many nutrients if it did not have so many tiny bumps. Whatever cannot be absorbed, the small intestine passes into the large intestine. There any extra water and salts are absorbed. What is left begins to form into **feces**.

The Big Glands

Near the stomach lies the liver. In an adult the liver weighs more than 3 pounds (1 kg). It plays a part in digestion by making bile. This greenish yellow liquid is stored in the gallbladder. The gallbladder is a small pouch that is fixed to the bottom of the liver. The gallbladder releases bile into the small intestine. There bile helps break down fats. The pancreas is a large, yellow gland just below the stomach. It makes a digestive juice that is released into the small intestine.

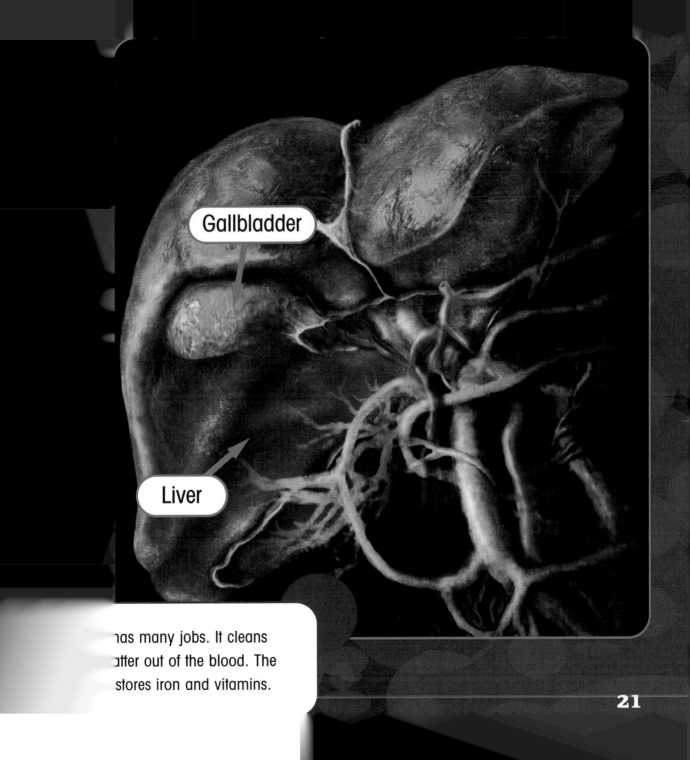

Gallbladder

Liver

...has many jobs. It cleans
...tter out of the blood. The
...stores iron and vitamins.

Digestive Trouble

Many things can go wrong in the digestive system. Some people's digestive systems have trouble breaking down certain parts of food, such as gluten. Gluten is a protein found in some breads. Many digestive problems are caused by not eating healthy food.

Our bodies work best when we get a lot of water and plenty of energy from fresh, vitamin-rich food. We should think about what we eat and the trip our food takes through the digestive system.

Glossary

acids (A-sidz) Liquids that break down matter faster than water does.

calories (KA-luh-reez) Amounts of food that the body uses to keep working.

carbohydrates (kar-boh-HY-drayts) What some foods, such as bread, are made of.

esophagus (ih-SAH-fuh-gus) A tunnel that ties the pharynx to the stomach.

feces (FEE-seez) What leaves your body as waste.

gastric juice (GAS-trik JOOS) An acid that your body uses to break down food.

glands (GLANDZ) Body parts that make liquids that help break down food into energy. Some glands also help take away waste from the body.

jaw (JAH) Bones in the top and bottom of the mouth.

liquid (LIH-kwed) Matter that moves like water.

lungs (LUNGZ) The parts of an air-breathing animal that take in air and supply oxygen to the blood.

minerals (MIN-rulz) Matter found in nature that is not an animal, a plant, or another living thing.

muscle (MUH-sul) A part of the body that is used to make the body move.

nutrients (NOO-tree-ints) Food that a living thing needs to live and grow.

pharynx (FA-rinks) A tunnel of muscle that ties the mouth to the tunnels leading to the lungs and the stomach.

proteins (PROH-teenz) Important parts of the cells of all plants and animals.

tongue (TUNG) A group of muscles inside the mouth.

vitamins (VY-tuh-minz) Nutrients that help the body fight illness and grow strong.

Index

A
acids, 4, 8, 16

B
bones, 8, 11

C
calorie, 7
carbohydrates, 8

E
energy, 7–8
esophagus, 16

F
fats, 8, 20

G
gallbladder, 20

gastric juices, 16
glands, 11, 16
gums, 12

L
large intestine, 19
liver, 20

M
minerals, 8
mouth, 11–12, 15
muscle(s), 4, 8,
    11, 15, 19

N
nutrients, 4, 19

P
pancreas, 20
pharynx, 15
proteins, 4, 8, 16

S
saliva, 11, 15
small intestine, 16,
    19–20
stomach, 16, 20
swallowing, 15

T
teeth, 11–12
tongue, 11, 15

V
vitamins, 8

Web Sites

Due to the changing nature of Internet links, PowerKids Press has developed an online list of Web sites related to the subject of this book. This site is updated regularly. Please use this link to access the list: www.powerkidslinks.com/hybw/digestive/